AF798081

SCHOOL OF HEIGHT

A.S. Palko

SCHOOL OF HEIGHT

A compilation of articles first appearing in the

Fitness and Sports Review International

Translated by Dr. Michael Yessis

Published by:

Ultimate Athlete Concepts

Michigan USA

2007

For information and to order copies: www.ultimateathleteconcepts.com

Part I - General Preparation

An article titled "So You Want To Grow a Little?" was published in Legkaya Atletika a few months ago. It discussed a widespread problem: how you can increase your height and whether it's generally possible. The editors promised a series by Orthopedist Anatoly Palko describing his methods.

Nature, as it were, has "programmed" each person, including a height or growth program. Many studies of short adults have shown they could have been taller, but they didn't reach their potential.

The reasons are many. An infection, a seeming insignificant injury, a vitamin deficiency, an inflammation—all of these can interfere with a child or teenager's bone development. They can also hamper one's growth-period nutrition.

The spinal cord grows in spurts, unevenly. Girls grow rapidly from the age of 10 to 14; boys, from 13 to 18. If negative factors are present during these years, growth slows down or halts. To recapture what was lost is difficult.. Spinal-cord growth and the growth of long tubular bones are influenced by both internal factors and by external stimuli during the growth period. The positive stimuli include: exercises for specific muscle groups, deep muscle massage, Circulation-enhancing hydrothermal therapy, work on training machines, hardening (getting the body accustomed to adverse conditions), physiotherapy, auto-training, and well-balanced nutrition. In addition, hypophysis-produced hormones are important.

Nicotine is one of the worst growth inhibitors. It suppresses the hypophysis, causes vascular spasms, and slows down the metabolism. As a result, growth-period nutrition worsens. Followers of our methods should draw the obvious conclusion about smoking. Here are the main factors inhibiting one from achieving his potential growth.

Don't think that doing certain exercises (such as jumping exercises or horizontal bar hangs) and enrolling in a class is enough. In reality it's much more complicated. First, you must follow the designated regimen and carry out all of our recommendations. Often I am asked what's primary and what's secondary (to save time). Our system contains no superfluous, secondary exercises or activities. It's important to follow our sequence of recommended activities. We use training machine workouts and all of the previously mentioned methods as tools to increase height. However, you should carefully prepare your muscles, joints, and ligaments before starting training machine workouts in order to avoid undue discomfort. As a first priority you should increase your range of movement and flexibility. Pay particular attention to the lumbar and hip areas. Your networking muscles should be fully relaxed and your working muscles tense when you perform the exercises.

Persistence, will power, purposefulness and workout consistency are all necessary to achieve best results.

Beware of a common error. Many people desiring growth hang for hours on a horizontal bar, constantly increasing the weight attached to their legs; alas, results don't appear, even though you would think that the spinal column would be stretched.

This method simply doesn't stimulate growth. On the contrary, the heavy resistance weight stimulates tension and contraction in the powerful trunk muscles. These muscles should be relaxed so the spinal column can be stretched by stretching the intervertebral disks. When we remove tension from the muscle (via massage and heat therapy), the blood supply improves and stimulates growth zones.

Let's begin with gymnastics. Our exercises are of medium difficulty. With them you prep the muscles for more advanced flexibility exercises. You should increase the load gradually, depending on your fitness level. We'll make the assignment more difficult with each workout. We'll start working on training machines when the muscles and joints become supple, flexible, pliable.

EXERCISES

1. Initial position (IP): standing, legs foot-width apart, with arms extended overhead and clasped together. Rise up on your toes and vigorously stretch upward; then drop your arms and clasp your hands behind your back and stand on your heels and raise your toes. Repeat 10-12 times.

2. IP: standing, with your legs foot-width apart, with arms to the side. Rotate forward alternately in the wrist, elbow, and shoulder joints. Repeat 10-12 times. Lower your arms, relax, and repeat the movement in the opposite direction.

3. IP: standing, with legs shoulder-width apart. Tilt your head to the right and left. Try to touch your ear to your shoulder (without lifting the shoulder). Repeat 10-12 times in each direction

4. IP: standing, with legs wider than the shoulders. Bend forward, touching the fingers (palms) to the floor. Repeat 20 times.

5. IP: standing, with feet shoulder-width apart. Arch backward, trying to touch the heels with the fingers. Repeat 20 times.

6. IP: standing, with the right leg bent at the knee and the foot pressed against the left knee. Bend forward, touching the fingers to the floor. Repeat 10 times on each leg.

7. IP: draw the arms backward and grip a cross-bar or the back of a chair (around shoulder-blade level). Squat while not letting go with the arms. Repeat 20 times.

8. IP: standing, with legs together. Bend forward, touching the forehead to the knees. Repeat 20 times.

9. IP: sitting on the floor, with one leg straight and forward and the other leg bent at the knee with the foot pulled backward. Bend forward, touching the floor with the arms. Repeat 20 times.

10. IP: lying on your back, with legs outstretched and arms to the side. Alternate lifting each leg until a right angle is formed.

11. IP: lying on your abdomen, with legs straight and arms straight along the body. Lift your head, shoulders and legs and clasp your legs with your arms and pull upward.

12. IP: kneeling, with support on the arms, which are placed shoulder-width apart. Bend forward while simultaneously sitting on your heels. Touch the floor with outstretched arms and drop your head.

13. IP: sitting, on your heels and arms clasped in front of yourself. Lift your arms and stretch upward as high as possible.

14. IP: sitting on the floor, with legs extended forward. Bend forward, touching the ends of your toes with your hands and touching your knees with your head.

15. IP: lying on your back, with arms at the waist. Gradually lift your legs upward and try to "throw" them behind your head.

Repeat exercises 10 through 15 for 15-20 repetitions.

Part II - Flexibility Development

In the previous article I provided a set of exercises that you should include in your morning exercises, if you've mastered them. In this article we'll study more advanced exercises. These loosen the spine, strengthen spinal and trunk muscles, enhance coordination, increase the range of movement and lengthen the spine (including the cervical portion). These exercises increase height and foster correct posture.

You should pay special attention to posture because it influences height significantly. The more your spine sags, the shorter your height. When your muscles are weak, the spinal column, as it were, "sits"; this loss of height can be as much as 10 centimeters. A small amount of spinal curvature may be justified, but it mustn't exceed the allowable limits: cervical spine" 2-2.5 centimeters; lower spine, 2.53.0 centimeters (you can check this by standing and pressing your spine to the wall). When you've attained correct posture, i.e., are able to touch the wall at five points (heels, calves, buttocks, spine, and back of the head), remember this position. Deliberately control yourself until correct posture becomes a habit.

Do not attack this set of exercises until you've mastered the first ones. You can work out at any convenient time except during the 1.5-2.0 hours after meals. We recommend you not work out when you're overfatigued or when you have a chronic or acute illness.

EXERCISES

1. Initial position (IP): sitting on the floor, with legs apart. Bend your right leg at the knee until the heel touches the crotch. Bend your left leg and position it so that the outer side of the foot touches the right knee. Rotate your trunk to the left and grip your left foot with your right hand. After turning further to the left,

place your left arm behind the back and touch the right hip. Turn your head so that your chin is above the left shoulder (Figure 1).

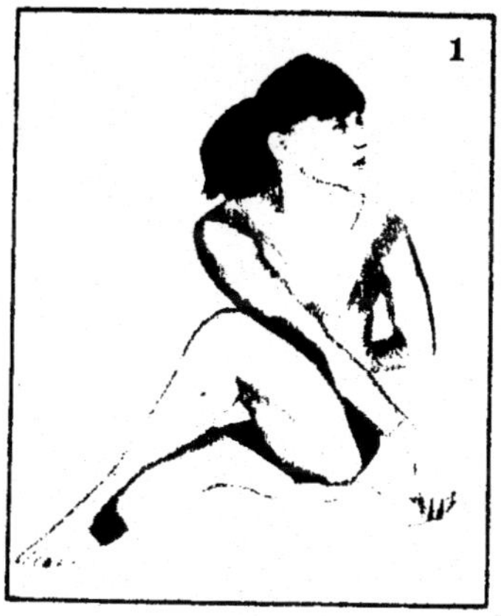

Rotate the trunk, shoulder, and head while inhaling slowly and deeply. Hold this position for a few seconds while holding your breath. Then return to the starting position while exhaling, making no sharp movements.

The final movement is sliding the right arm from the foot to the knee of the left leg while leaning the trunk backward. Return to the initial position and relax.

Repeat twice in both directions.

2. IP: standing, with legs together. Lift your arms overhead, take a deep breath, and slowly bend forward. Touch your toes with your hands, and touch your knees with your nose. Exhale. Hold this position for 5 seconds. Return to the starting position and inhale. Repeat 4 times.

3. IP: lying on your abdomen. After inhaling slowly and deeply, lift your head as high as you can. Then tense your back muscles and elevate your shoulders; tilt your trunk backward, supporting yourself with your arms. Hold your breath and maintain this position for 7-12 seconds. Then exhale slowly and return to the starting position.

4. IP: lying on your back, with muscles relaxed. Slowly lift the legs until they form a 90 degree angle with the trunk. While supporting yourself on your arms and elbows, go into a stand on your forearms and remain in this position for

3-4 minutes (later, up to 10 minutes); then return to the starting position and

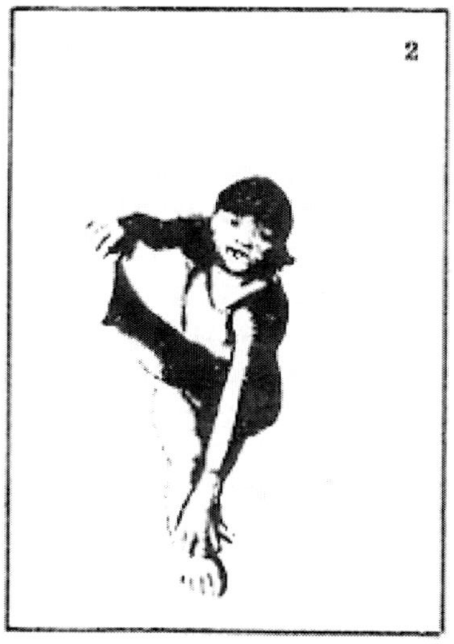

5. IP: sitting on the floor with your legs extended in front of you. Grasp the toes of your left foot with your right hand and lift upward as high as you can. The left arm should be touching the right foot. Hold this position for 1-2 minutes. Your breathing should consciously be slow, and deep (Figure 2).

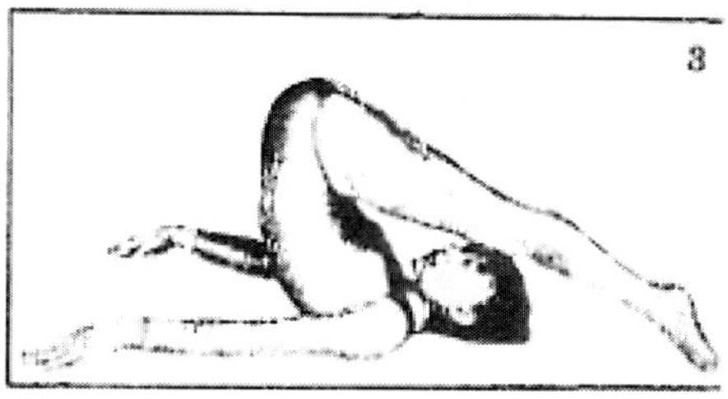

6. IP: lying on your back with arms slightly to the side and palms down. Lift your legs upward to a 45 degree angle and then, after a pause, to a right angle. Your breathing should be slow and deep. Bring your legs behind your head and hold this position for several seconds. Then drop them slowly behind your head, touching your toes to the floor, with the knees straight (Figure 3). Breathe deeply.

Extend the legs still further. Bend the knees as much as possible and touch them to your head. Remain in this position for a few seconds until fatigue sets in. Then return slowly to the starting position.

7. IP: standing, with legs apart, arms to the side at shoulder level, palms down. Bend slowly to the left, trying to reach your hand to your foot. Hold this position 5 seconds and then return slowly to the starting position. Repeat twice in both directions. Your breathing should be deliberate.

8. IP: lying on your stomach, with your legs together. Bend your elbows and position at shoulder level with palms down. Elevate your trunk as high as you can. Tilt your head backward. Breathing should be deliberate and through the nose.

Turn to the left so that you can see your right heel (leave your legs and arms in place and keep the lower part of your stomach on the floor); then turn to your right so that you can see your left heel. Again arch upward and backward and drop down to the starting position.

Repeat, using the sequence "up-right-left-down" and hold each position for 2-30 seconds.

9. IP: sitting in a squatting position with your arms clasped in front of you. Then drop your head along with your locked fingers so that the parietal region touches the floor.

Pull up your knees slowly. Push off the floor and lift your legs upward until they are fully extended. Hold this position for 5-20 seconds (Figure 4). Then return slowly to the starting position, stand up straight and stand for 1-2 minutes in order to recover your normal blood circulation.

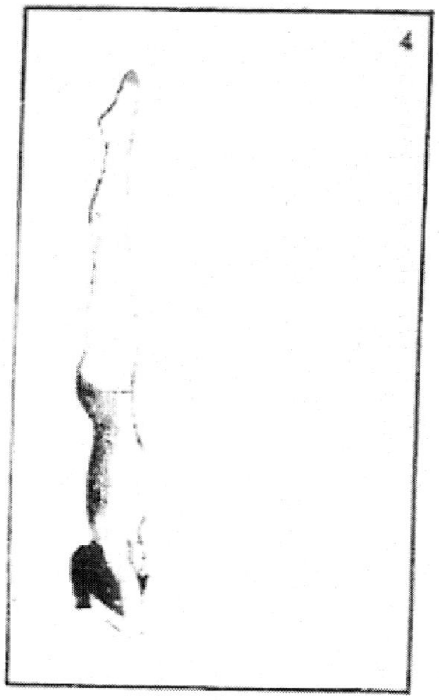

You can use spotters when working with these exercises. Breathe through your nose.

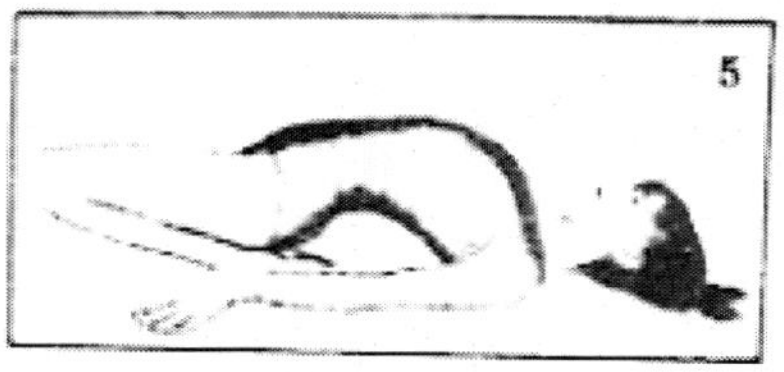

10. IP: sitting on heels. Throw your head backward and lean backward slowly, touching the crown to the floor, with the arms extended along the trunk (Figure 5). Hold this position for 1-2 minutes. Breathe deeply and slowly.
Return to the starting position, keeping your hands on the floor.

Part III—Asymmetric Exercises

In this installment we'll acquaint you with a training aid you should use diligently. It consists of two pulleys, spaced some distance from each other and spanned by a cable. A weight (not more than one-third of the user's body weight) hangs from one end of the cable; the other end of the cable attaches to a horizontal bar (you can use a gymnastic stick). Any sort of pulley will do. The set-up can be installed in a doorway (Fig 1) or in a corner of a room (Fig 2).

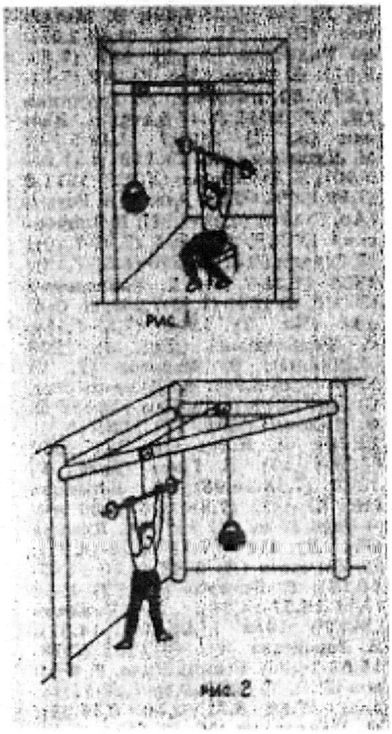

Before you work out on this device you should master another type of gymnastic exercise. It's important to reach certain goals or indexes, but it's also important to maintain them. Not everyone succeeds in doing the latter. Some people have increased their height several centimeters by using the training machine but have then lost the increase after a certain period of time. The reason was a habitual motor pattern relating to their posture.

Conditioned reflexes are typical of the trunk muscles, which function automatically. It's fairly complex to change them. Changing them requires new, unfamiliar interrelationships between the different muscle groups. It's not easy to restructure the voluntary conditioned reflexes, so we have put together special exercises— called "asymmetric exercises"—for this purpose.

Rhythm forms the basis of each movement. This type of exercise combines the various rhythms and movements of symmetric body parts. These exercises first develop the skill to control and accomplish several movements simultaneously.

Systematic workouts teach one to exceed the limits of conditioned reflexes. Having internal control and adapting easily to rhythm changes makes it happen.

You should include these exercises in your daily workouts. You can do them immediately after the exercises we covered previously in this series or you can do them separately before workouts on the training device. Do all exercises first to the right and then to the left, for 10-15 repetitions.

EXERCISES

1. Starting position: standing with arms extended in front. Make circles with one hand and equilateral triangles with the other. The count is optional.

2. Starting position: standing or sitting, arms in front of the chest, elbows bent, and palms down. Rotate one arm clockwise, slightly extending it at the elbow joint; rotate the other counterclockwise.

3. Starting position: standing. Make clockwise circles with your arm extended in front. Simultaneously, make counterclockwise circles with the wrist of the same hand. Perform the movements smoothly without jerks and keep the elbow straight. After finishing the exercise with one arm, do it with both arms.

4. Starting position: Make a loud clap overhead and strike the floor softly with the leg. Change the force of the footstrike using a count of five. Finish the exercise with a slight overhead clap and a strong footstrike.

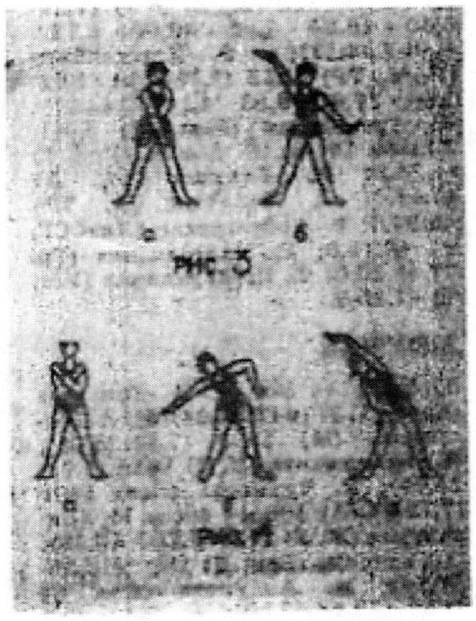

5. Starting position: standing with feet shoulder-width apart. On a count of "one" the arms are straight and crossed as in Fig 3a; on a count of "two" the right arm is straight and overhead (open palm facing upward) and the left arm is downward (palm facing down) as in Fig 3b; on a count of "three" the hands are made into fists; on a count of "four" both wrists are at a right angle to the forearm; on a count of "five" the arms are crossed, hanging down, with fists clenched; on the count of "six" you change the arm position.

6. Starting position: standing, with feet shoulder-width apart. On the count of "one" cross the arms on the chest (Fig 4a); on the count of "two" let the right arm drop down and bend the trunk to the right lifting the left arm toward the shoulder and bending the elbow (Fig 4b); on the count of "three" lift the left arm, taking it straight overhead, and lower the right shoulder with the right elbow slightly bent (Fig 4c).

7. Starting position: lying on your left side. On the count of "one" bend the legs, forming right angles at the knees; the right arm is overhead, while the left lies on the floor. On the count of "two" turn, using the trunk and leg muscles; change the arm position— place the right arm on your torso.

8. Starting position: lying on your back, legs straight. On a count of "one" bend the right leg at the hip and knee joints, arms behind your head, lift the trunk and turn to the right. On the count of "two" change the leg position and rotate the trunk to the left.

9. Starting position: lying, turn onto your right side and rise up, legs together, while supported on your right arm. On the count of "one" extend the left leg as far as possible at the hip joint and bend the knee joint, grasping it with the hand and bringing it as close to the trunk as possible (Fig 5a). On the count of "two" bend the leg at the hip and knee, grasp it behind the foot and bring it as close to the trunk as possible (Fig 5b).

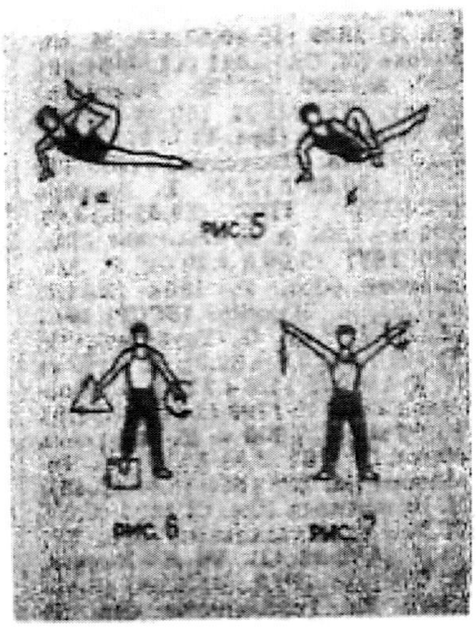

10. Starting position: seated on the floor, With legs apart, with the left arm hanging down alongside the trunk, with the right arm behind the head. The arms should be straight. On the count of "one" grasp a leg with the arms and lean the torso toward the floor. On the count of "two" lean the torso forward and bend the arms. On the count of "three" grasp the second leg with the hands and bend the torso. On the count of "four" bring the legs together, grasp the torso with the arms and move closer to the floor.

11. Starting position: standing, legs foot-width apart, arms spread a little to the side. Inscribe a triangle with the right hand and a circle with the left hand. Simultaneously inscribe a square (Fig 6) with the foot).

12. Starting position: standing, legs shoulder-width apart, arms apart and to the side, pointed slightly upward. Move the right arm up and down and inscribe a circle with the left arm (Fig 7).

You need preparatory training for most of these exercises even if you've trained previously.

Part IV - Nutrition and Height

In this article we'll discuss nutrition for those who want to increase their growth/height. Our workouts require extra physical and mental energy and require top quality building material. Nutritional indiscretions can, in themselves, be one of the reasons for retarded growth.

First, it's imperative to maintain a balance of proteins, fats, carbohydrates, vitamins, minerals, and other nutritionally relevant substances.

Nutritional variations can and should be diverse, but we should avoid erroneous experiments on our own bodies, especially the extremes that are promoted by incompetent people. Pure vegetarianism, raw-foodism, fruitarianism, flower eating, and excessive use of honey may turn out to be ineffective means of increasing growth and may be dangerous to health. The reason for this is that there's no consideration for individual differences in a person's constitution, living conditions, and activity.

We recommend you use a wide variety of vegetable and animal products, but subject them to minimal cooking. This helps to preserve their biological activity.

Experts recommend that we use fresh fruits and vegetables 3-4 times a day (2-3 types - about 1.5 kg per day). Vegetables are very important in human nutrition. They should be a part of our diet year around. Spicy-tasting and perennial greens occupy an important place. This category includes the following vegetables, which vary biologically and nutritionally: leafy and cabbage salads, spinach, watercress, leafy parsley and celery, dill, perennial onions, rhubarb, asparagus, and tarragon.

These plants are rich in vitamins, minerals, and contain proteins, carbohydrates, and organic acids. There's a lot of vitamin C in green vegetables. The minerals contained in these plants (potassium, sodium, calcium, etc.) perform an important metabolic function.

From the earliest of times man has used both wild and cultivated plants as food. From early in spring they've supplied vitamins. In lean crop years they've substituted for bread in the summer and fall. Many wild perennial grasses that grow in our country contain a wide array of biologically active substances. Individual samples of wild flora are often richer in these compounds then cultivated plants. Examples are nettle, orach, dandelion, plantain, mint, coltsfoot, kislitsa (name for acid-tasting grasses), rose-bay, willow-herb, borage, the common sow-thistle, and many more. We'll give you some recipes. However, if you want to know more about nutrition in today's environment and how to utilize naturally occurring plants, we recommend Choosing Health (Mikhailov, Palko, Young Guard Press, 1985).

You can harvest wild edible plants from early spring to late autumn. We don't recommend you collect plants in a city within 500 meters of a street or railroad track because plants assimilate and accumulate lead and other harmful substances from automobile exhaust. You should collect young juicy sprouts and leaves. Wash them carefully and pour boiling water over them before using them raw.

The warm part of the year is an opportune time to provide yourself with optimal nutrition and prepare for winter. Growth is not accomplished in a mere couple of months. You have to devote a lot of time to it.

Extensive use of vegetable and animal products helps normalize metabolism and body mass, and increase vital activity.

A sound nutritional regimen increases growth by about 10 percent in all people, independent of their constitution (of course they have to follow all of the methods and recommendations that are designed to increase growth). Alcohol and smoking should be avoided completely.

Grains are good growth stimulators. You should give priority to black bread and various cooked grains.

Here are a few recipes:

Buttered bread and greens

Mash 100 grams of butter, salt it, and add 2-3 tablespoons of finely chopped parsley greens or other greens and a teaspoon of lemon juice. Whip the entire mixture and spread in on a slice of bread.

Flatcakes with beets

Mix one-half cup flour with one-half cup semolina. Wash 3 beets and 2 apples, run them through a mincing machine, and mix with the flour and semolina. Into this mixture pour 10 grams of yeast dissolved in warm water and let stand for 30-45 minutes. Then add 2 tablespoons of chopped nettle and orach. Salt to taste. Make flat-cakes of 50-100 grams from the resulting mixture and place them on a dry griddle. Bake in oven 20-30 minutes, then spread with butter.

Kasha from mixed groats

Without mixing, wash 2 tablespoons of rice, pearl barley, wheat and buckwheat. Clean 3-4 carrots, cut them into sticks and place in the bottom of a saucepan (fifth part). Then spread layers of carrots, wheat, carrots, pearl barley, carrots, buckwheat, and carrots. Pour over 2 cups of cold water, bring to a boil and boil thoroughly for 10-15 minutes. Salt to taste. Then let stand under cover for 20-30 minutes without mixing. Pour in 1 glass of mile and bring to a boil. Remove from heat and add 3 tablespoons butter.

Soup

Clean 3-5 potatoes, cut them into thin circles, pour in 1 liter of hot bone broth, cook 5-7 minutes and then let stand for 10-15 minutes. Salt to taste. Place into the prepared potatoes 2 cut carrots, 2 tomatoes, 2 Bulgarian peppers (including seeds), 1 large onion head, 2 tablespoons of finely chopped raspberry leaves, 1 table-spoon of finely chopped orach, and 2 bay leaves.

Fruit-vegetable combo with tea

Clean and cut into sticks 2 beets, 1 carrot, and 2 apples. Mix with 4 tablespoons of jam or preserves. Pour in one glass of water. Add one-quarter teaspoon of citric acid or the juice of *a* lemon and a little vanilla. Mix in 1 tablespoon of finely chopped raspberry leaves, mints, nettles, and black currants. Then boil the mixture thoroughly for 5-6 minutes, cool, and add to the tea.

Cottage cheese with nettle

Put 200 grams of cottage cheese through a sieve and mix with it 1 cup of finely chopped nettle leaves and young sprouts (washed carefully beforehand), 3 cloves of finely chopped garlic, 1 teaspoon of mustard and 3 tablespoons of vegetable oil.

Broth of diclinous nettle leaves

Dip 15 grams of nettle leaves in 1 cup of boiling water and let stand for 10 minutes. Drink one-third of a cup 3 times a day. This drink contains carotene and vitamins C and K, among others.

Broth of dogrose fruits

Crush 1 tablespoon of dogrose fruits, pour on 2 cups of boiling water and boil thoroughly on a double boiler for 15-20 minutes. Let it stand for a day and run through a strainer. Consume one-half cup 2 times a day.

You can use these dishes 2-3 times a week. We'll introduce you to other recipes that will help you make the transition to sound nutrition while you're working at increasing your growth.

Part V - Pressure Massage

I hope you have already mastered the general conditioning exercises, flexibility exercises, and asymmetric exercises that we have discussed in previous installments. Additionally, we have discussed the topic of nutrition.

In this installment we focus on massage, but not conventional massage. This different type of massage uses rugs with pins or needles. First let us cover some history and some general concepts concerning human skin and its functions.

The notion of the skin serving a primitive function has been replaced by fundamental research showing conclusively that human skin is very active and is just a important as any other organ. Our external shield has one unique capacity- the capacity to respond not only at the spot where it is stimulated, but in different organs and systems, and to restore or strengthen functional capacities.

It is no accident that folk medicine men of the East have dubbed skin the "big parade door" through which pathological conditions come and go.

Physicians in all continents noted sensitive locations to which to apply a stimulus in order to achieve a desired result. Some of the various methods used are: rubbing, pressing, massage, pricking, searing, and cauterization. In the East they have used needles of rock, of bone, and of metal. In ancient Egypt they used agents such as Spanish fly (Cantharides) plasters, mustard plasters, fomentations of copper vitriol, alcohol and even artificial aseptic inflammations. Mongolians in Corsica and Arabia have used red-hoot iron, stones, hot oil or other fats for the same purposes.

The world-wide spread of acupuncture has undeservedly pushed some of these simple methods of stimulating reflex zones into the background. In contrast with acupuncture-which should only be done by a specialist—these methods can be used independently.

What is the secret of effectively using these primitive methods on human skin?

The skin is our most sensitive system. It is like a sensor aimed at the external world which—via numerous links—communicates with all organs and tissues through the central nervous system. One square centimeter of skin has about 150 pain receptors, 25 tactile receptors, 12 cold receptors, and 2 heat receptors.

We have recorded about 700 points having a therapeutic value. In addition, there are about 20 "forbidden" points where stimulation can be harmful. That is why we follow specialists' recommendations so as to get the maximum, benefit from the skin's sanitary, stimulating and therapeutic qualities. For our purposes we only need to know the most important points and some zones where we can generally reap a benefit.

Hand and foot massage are important. In the opinion of many investigators, the hands and feet are like a switchboard containing over a hundred thousand "switching" points; we can stimulate any part of the body by acting on them. Most of us rub our hands when we have to do something important on the spur of the moment. Plato wrote that walking barefooted not only toughens one, but sharpens one's thoughts. The Spartans outlawed the use of footwear before the age of 18.

In the last several decades man has become less active and more sedentary. Skin is being shielded and sealed off by clothing and footwear. Contact with the surrounding world is becoming more and more meager. Many important adaptations fade away from prolonged inactivity, and this a surely has an effect on all indices of activity.

We developed and are proposing a method of stimulation massage using a rug with plastic needles and/or pins. However, if your skin is delicate and pressure massage (i.e., pressure on many points) causes pain or produces persistent difficulties, you can do the initial sessions on a rubber rug having pins that are sold in a domestics store. Various plastic forms are used today, so it is easy to choose and construct your own massager. When choosing a surface, seek out "fat" plastic materials; they slide along stretched skin more easily and do not inflict injury.

Use the rugs only for massage, and keep them clean and dry in a polyethylene package.

Massage is contraindicated when there are infections and illnesses requiring surgery. You should not massage warts, birthmarks, dirty skin or inflamed skin containing lesions, or varicose veins.

Pressure massage should not last more than 15 minutes.

Before you massage a body part you should wash it with soap and warm water and then cover it with vaseline that has been warmed in your hand. Stroke, rub, and knead the selected areas before and after the massage session.

Loosen any tight clothing before doing the exercises. Avoid sharp movements. Do pressure massage as a separate procedure or combine it with exercises.

Do not be distracted during the massage. Listen to your body's feelings.

EXERCISES

1. Starting position: sitting, with feet on the rug. Get up and stand for 1 minute. Do the exercises 3-5 times.

2. Starting position: sitting on a chair, with your feet on the rug. Move onto the balls of your feet, then roll onto your heels, gradually increasing the pressure on your foot. Do this 10-15 times. This exercise lets you waken faster from sleep, and it stimulates internal organs.

3. Starting position: standing in front of the rug. Rise on the rug, alternating your left and right feet, and stand 1 minute. Do 2-3 times with each leg.

4. Starting position: lying on your spine (rug under the spine). Lie and relax for 2-3 minutes.

5. Starting position: lying on your back (rug under the spine), hands on the floor and outstretched to the side, holding 2-10 kg. dumbbells (depending on your fitness level). Slowly lift the dumbbells upward and hold this position 1 minute.

6. Starting position: sitting on the floor with your knees pressed to your chest and your arms around them (place the rug so that it is under the spine during the roll). Do 4-10 backward rolls. This exercise improves blood circulation in the spinal area and reduces pain in cases of spinal myositis, lumbalgia, allergies, and osteochondrosis.

7. With the rug pressed in your hand, massage extra sensitive areas with increasingly intense vibration-like movements. This exercise reduces unpleasant sensations and lowers the pain threshold. You can use it several times a day.

8. Starting position: lying support (push-up) position (rug under the arms). Push off 3-10 times.

9. Starting position: sitting on your knees, lowered on to the heels, feet turned inward and crossed, arms supported in front of yourself (rug in front). Lift the knees, grasp the rug with your hands and push it under the knees (maximum pin pressure should be on the lower-outer edge of the patella) and lift the arms upward. Stay in this position 1 -3 minutes.

When compared with other methods, pressure massage fares well in its accessibility, effectiveness, and simplicity. Wit it you can relieve excess tension and increase physical activity. Pressure massage is an important tool for increasing growth and developing the body's capabilities.
In our next installment we will discuss autotraining.

Part VI - Breathing and Autogenic Training

In previous installments I've emphasized that it's important to follow our recommendations and be persistent and purposeful. That's why this installment concerns how—with the help of breathing and autogenic training—to relieve tension at the end of a workday and how to orient oneself to perform the exercises most effectively.

First let's talk about BREATHING and why it's so important. Your lungs contain about 700 million alveoli, the total area of which amounts to 100 sq/m. The alveoli are the main source of oxygen, the supplier of vital energy, and the place where carbon dioxide, the final product of oxidation is excreted.

Breathing is the sum total of all organic processes, including conversions that secrete quantum en/Kgy for biological reactions. Correct breathing helps to stimulate one or another body function. The cortex plays a critical role in regulating breathing, and every person possesses a remarkable capacity— the capacity to voluntarily control one's breathing.

We distinguish two types of breathing depending on the relative duration on inhalation and exhalation: mobilizing and sedative. Sedative breathing involves longer exhalation; stimulating breathing involves longer inhalation. By type, breathing should be diaphragmatic (abdominal). To avoid hyperventilation, include a short pause.

It is best to learn respiratory exercises while lying down, but it is possible while sitting. During the first sessions place your hand on your stomach; in this way you can control your breathing so that it's diaphragmatic. You should do breathing exercises with a stopwatch or by counting mentally.

If rhythm is disrupted, stop the activity and breathe voluntarily until automatic breathing normalizes. Then repeat the entire set of exercises.

For learning purposes, we show the cycle of breathing movements as fractions.

The numerator stands for the length of inhalation, the denonimator— the length of exhalation; the number in parentheses stands for the length of pause. During the first sessions, choose your own count. You shouldn't lengthen or shorten it; it's better to slow *it down or speed it up.*

SEDATIVE BREATHING

The first stage involves longer exhalation:

$\frac{4}{4+(2)}$ $\frac{4}{5+(2)}$ $\frac{4}{6+(2)}$ $\frac{4}{7+(2)}$ $\frac{4}{8+(2)}$

The second stage involves slightly longer inhalation and exhalation:

$\frac{4}{9+(2)}$ $\frac{5}{9+(2)}$ $\frac{5}{10+(2)}$

The third stage involves gradually longer inhalation, equaling exhalation at the end. With the deeper breathing, the pause lengthens somewhat:

$\frac{6}{110 + (3)}$ $\frac{7}{10 + (3)}$ $\frac{8}{10 + (4)}$ $\frac{9}{10 + (4)}$ $\frac{10}{10 + (5)}$

In the fourth stage the breathing cycle normalizes, but inhalation shortens:

$\frac{9}{10 + (4)}$ $\frac{8}{9+(4)}$ $\frac{7}{8+(3)}$ $\frac{6}{7+(3)}$ $\frac{5}{6+(2)}$

$\frac{4}{5 + (2)}$ $\frac{3}{4 + (2)}$

STIMULATING BREATHING

Stimulating breathing— in distinction from sedative breathing— involves a pause after inhalation.

In the first stage, inhalation is deeper and more energetic:

$\frac{4 + (2)}{4}$ $\frac{5 + (2)}{4}$ $\frac{5 + (2)}{4}$ $\frac{6 + (3)}{5}$ $\frac{7 + (3)}{5}$

In the second stage the entire breathing cycle lengthens:

$\frac{8+ (4)}{5}$ $\frac{9 + (4)}{5}$ $\frac{10+ (5)}{5}$

In the third stage, exhalation becomes gradually equal with inhalation:

$\frac{10+ (5)}{6}$ $\frac{10+ (5)}{7}$ $\frac{10+ (5)}{8}$ $\frac{10+ (5)}{9}$

$\frac{10+ (5)}{10}$ $\frac{10+ (5)}{10}$

In the fourth stage breathing returns to normal:

$\frac{10+(5)}{9}$ $\frac{9+(4)}{8}$ $\frac{8+(4)}{6}$ $\frac{7+(3)}{7}$ $\frac{6+(3)}{5}$

$\frac{5+(2)}{4}$ $\frac{4+(2)}{4}$

You've probably noticed that stimulating and sedative breathing are almost mirror images of each other.

Two weeks are enough to learn these types of breathing. It's best to practice in the fresh air or in a well ventilated room. The skill of controlling breathing can be used in various activities. Use mobilizing (stimulating) breathing if you need to reduce fatigue, drowsiness, or sluggishness. If, on the other hand, you need to calm yourself or reduce excess emotional tension or physical tension, use sedative breathing. It promotes deeper muscle relaxation, which is particularly valuable during autogenic training and during workouts for increasing flexibility.

AUTOGENIC TRAINING

No one denies that the first step toward success in any undertaking is a success-oriented psychology, and absolute confidence—at both the conscious and subconscious levels—in the correctness of one's actions. This is of no small importance when pursuing increased growth or height. According to domestic and foreign research data, using goal-directed active consciousness is a powerful resource for tapping the body's physical reserves. Such consciousness also forms the foundation for developing the skill of controlling certain bodily processes.

By concentrating your inner volitional attention, you may attain the necessary results in a shorter time period and with great effect. Autogenic training, which is a scientific psychological discipline based on autosuggestion, allows one, via complex psychic processes (mostly imaging, concentration, and emotional conditions), to influence organs that are normally autonomic and outside conscious control.

Every person can overcome objective and subjective obstacles arising enroute to goals by having desire, by being aware of what's essential, and by believing in one's own powers. Autosuggestion is effective when one lacks confidence, when one is overcoming and giving up bad habits, and when one is forming new skills.

One of the first skills one must master is the ability to consciously control muscle tone. First, the flow of CNS impulses declines when you reach full muscle relaxation. These impulses are freed up for increasing the level of other nerve processes, in particular, m for forming new connections. Second, and just as important, there's the skill or relaxing trunk muscles that work statically.

We can divide all muscles into two groups: muscles that work in a regime of short voluntary contractions and muscles that work under prolonged static tension. The later category includes the powerful muscle masses of the leg, the pelvic girdle, the trunk, the shoulder girdle, and the neck, which hold a person in a vertical position. Autogenic training and machine-aided training are necessary in order to control these muscle masses.

A person can attain complete muscle relaxation only if he possesses the skills of autotraining, which allows him to disengage all muscles from the motor centers of the cerebral cortex. We experience this condition of decreased tension as a rising feeling of deep rest, tranquility, and mild lassitude.

It is best to engage in autogenic training while lying down; however, one can master it while sitting. Autotraining is to be done immediately before working on training machines.

You should pay attention to body position. During sitting sessions, sit up straight in a chair with the spine straight. Then relax the muscles (do not bend forward), lower the head on the chest, spread the legs a little and bend them at an obtuse angle, place the arms on the knees, close the eyes, and relax the lower jaw (with mouth closed). This is the so-called active pose of Kuchera.

Passive postures are more comfortable, but they can be assumed in a soft chair that has an elbow rest or while lying in bed. Then the spinal column and the back of the head lies on the back edge of the chair or headrest, the arms rest on the armrests, and the rest of the position is the same; the toes should be pointed slightly to the side. The reclining position should be comfortable.

Before starting the session, tense and then relax your muscles. Focus your attention on the meaning of pronounced words (you can visualize yourself in the desired state); repeat each phrase 3-5 times. If success doesn't come immediately, don't despair. Sometimes 10 weeks are required among experienced specialists who are in an autotraining instruction course \that involves 1-1.5 hour daily workouts. After mastering the skill of dropping into a relaxed state, 5-10 minutes, and sometimes even less, is enough for autotraining. The text below isn't mandatory. You can choose your own; however, once it's chosen you shouldn't change it.

Pronounce all of the phrases mentally and don't be distracted by outside stimuli. Shut off the television and radio and isolate yourself from all outside noises. Pronounce the phrases slowly and listen to your body's reaction.

1. I'm quieting down. I'm perfectly calm.

2. My legs are getting heavy. My arms are becoming heavy.

3. Pleasant warmth is spreading into my left leg, gradually moving to my right leg, left arm, right arm. Warmth is spreading throughout my whole upper body.

4. My body is becoming warm.

5. My heart is beating softly.

6. My breathing is smooth and easy.

7. My upper body is relaxed.

8. My arm strength is being preserved and strengthened.

9. Workouts on the training machine (or for flexibility development) will be specially helpful. My body is being stretched maximally. It has become pliable and obedient.

During these phrases smoothly make your hands into fists and hold them in this position for 5-10 seconds 1 -2 times.

Afterward you can do a workout on a training machine (the training method will be published in the next installment).

Later on, when movements are automatic on the training machine, you can achieve the maximum effect by adding the following formula.

1. My entire body has become pliable.

2. It is getting longer and longer.

3. My upper body and legs are becoming longer.

4. I am growing slowly and steadily.

You should achieve greater muscle relaxation and pliability of the joint-ligament apparatus with each workout, and all of this should be reflected in increased growth and height.

I AM GROWING!! This thought should sink deep into your consciousness. You should concentrate your attention not only during autogenic training sessions, but all through the day.

Long layoffs from workouts are intolerable because they negatively affect measurements of growth increase. Mastering autogenic training simplifies the process of increasing growth and allows you to achieve the desired effect in less time.

Part VII - Training Aids

This installment is devoted to the use of training aids. However, before we start to explain methods, let's discuss some general questions associated with the problem of using weight-resistance exercise to increase height.

The literature contains articles which state that hanging from horizontal bars and with weight resistance helps increase height. However, I've accumulated many letters in which users of these methods say that they have not grown a single millimeter, despite the fact that daily they suspended themselves for hours from a horizontal bar, often with as much as 20 kg. attached to their legs. We will now try to sort out this contradiction.

A person's movement during various activities, including standing, and even sitting, requires continuous muscle tension to hold the trunk vertical. These massive muscle groups are located on top of the skeleton's joints and ligaments; it's as if an "armor" has been pulled as tight as a drawn bow over the skeleton, limiting its mobility. From the moment of arising from bed in the morning till going to bed at night, these muscles get no rest. Were this not the case, a person would simply lie prostrate on the ground.

The habitual motor pathways developed over the years, during a time in which the load on the body was increasing, induce "automatic" tension in these muscles, the greater part of which is controlled subconsciously. This is why most people build up muscle mass, instead of increasing their height, when they work on a horizontal bar.

The simply-constructed training aids we are proposing allow an athlete to develop the skill to control these muscles. Observations have shown that the more highly trained a person's ability to voluntarily relax muscle masses with static loads, the better his training results.

Why does a person's height increase during training?

Bones become longer, various deformations are eliminated, posture is improved, the elasticity of joint surfaces is restored, and, for those who are in the growing stage-the "growth zone" is stimulated.

I must disappoint those who, having missed our previous installments, put their faith in increasing height through the use of training aids. This erroneous notion generally leads to inferior training activities and insignificant results. You see, this displaced emphasis will allow other potentials of the human organism to remain untapped and unrealized. In previous installments we acquainted readers with some methods of developing flexibility, organizing an effective nutrition system, asymmetric gymnastics, and pressure-type massage, which are needed as preparation for using a training aid.

Activities designed to increase height should last at least 1 1/2-2 1/2 hours. The activities can be performed several times over the course of a day, as the person's daily regimen and life style allows. During a period of workouts designed to increase height, try to avoid strenuous physical workloads. An exemplary plan for structuring a workout could be as follows. After a light warm-up, do flexibility exercises; warm the muscles by using one of the passive methods (a heating pad, bath, shower, sauna); do pressure-type massage (which should be combined with autogenic training); then start using the training aids. Figures 1 and 2 show the structural details of the mechanical and spring-operated devices to use to increase height.

What training approach should be used with the training aids? During the first workouts, the trainee shouldn't suspend weight-or create a pulling force--of more than 20-25% of his body weight. The amount of weight should build up gradually and by the end of the first year it should reach 75-80% of the athlete's body weight. The following is a model plan for increasing the weight. If the athlete's body weight is 70 kg., the first weight should be 14-17 kg.; if he increases it by 150 gm a day (excluding the off days), it will reach 56-60 kg. by the end of the year.

Once again I want to repeat: training-aid workouts should be started with light resistance, which can be built up to the desired level in 3-4 sets. Here is why the spring-operated training aid with a scale (dynamometer) has an advantage over the training aid using a pulley and a weight. A specially constructed handle is used in the spring-operated training aid; a pulley winds around the handle, thereby controlling its length, and dispenses the effort throughout the workout. The movements should be done smoothly, rhythmically and slowly, to avoid sharp jerking motions.

The length of the pulley is controlled so that the athlete can grasp the crossbar at shoulder width with his outstretched arms by rising on his toes. The crossbar is best made in a triangular shape; it is more convenient for gripping, and when fatigue sets in it can be better kept from slipping. After gripping the crossbar, drop down flatfooted and lift the weight; on the spring-operated training aid, make sure the indicator is set at the required resistance.

If people of different heights train on the same device, use different sized blocks under the legs or mount a mechanism in the crossbar that allows the length of the cable to be changed smoothly.

During the first 10-12 workouts, the trainee needs to learn to relax (by 3-4 cm) the trunk muscles that are controlled by the pulley movement when the trunk is extended and the arms out stretched. Make sure that the movement in this exercise occurs solely as a result of the trunk lengthening, and not as a result of opening the fingers or rising onto the toes. In the first days, the work on the training aid should last 15-20 minutes; then daily add 3-5 minutes to bring the time to 11 /2-2 hours. If lumbar pain or discomfort appears, consult with a physician.

After the student has learned to relax his trunk muscles, he should perform a series of dampening (slowly extinguishing) exercises for range of motion and try to maximally elongate the body at the moment of "extinguishing" of the movement. These nonstationary fluctuations should be done in forward-backward, side-to-side and circular directions. In each case, a set lasts about 3-5 minutes. Between sets, take a rest, preferably lying down; and combine the rest with autogenic work.

For best results, don't allow yourself to become distracted; clearly plan the course of the session; don't carry on conversations with those around you. Focus your attention on your main goal-to increase your height. It is helpful to accompany the workout with soft music. For this purpose, use symphonic works or folk melodies with soft, slow rhythms.

The fluctuations in height during a workout may be within the range of 0.3-2 cm, depending on the athlete's idiosyncrasies, the intensity of the workout, and the time of day; moreover, the growth from individual workouts is not stable-it only lasts for several hours to a day or more. However, systematic workouts not only help maintain the level of growth; they also help it in crease steadily.

Again I would like to remind the reader: do workouts systematically; avoid long gaps between workouts.

The Mechanical
Training Aid

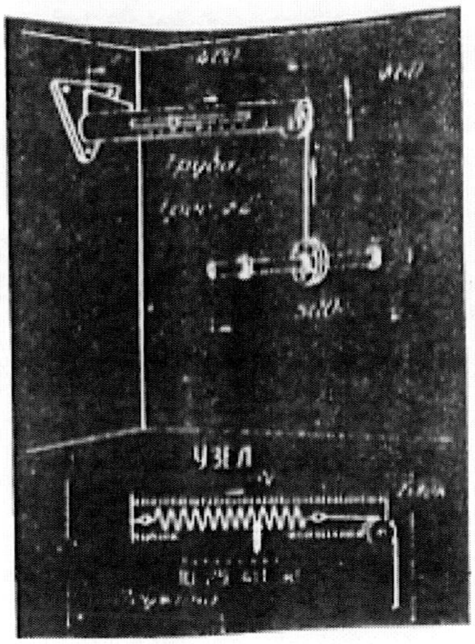

Fig.1

Resilient
Training Aie

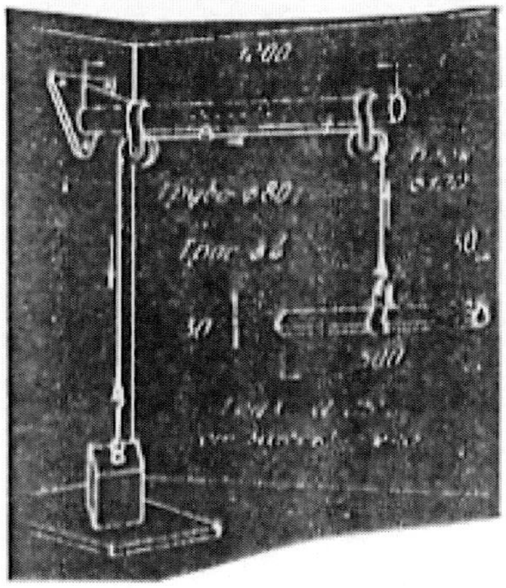

Fig.2